BEAT YOUR
LUPUS

The New Dietary Approach

SECOND EDITION

Exploring the Causes, Mechanism, and Treatment of Lupus

Steven A. Baranowitz, M.D.

Illustrations by Sidney Reyes

SECOND EDITION

ISBN: 978-0-9973044-0-4 (Paperback)
ISBN: 978-0-9973044-1-1 (eBook)

Printed in the United States of America

*This book is dedicated to my mother,
who realized there was a link between food and
autoimmune disease, long before her son became a
doctor.*

Preface

This book was written for Lupus patients and their families.

By reading this book, you will be able to:

- Gain new intelligent insight on how to beat your Lupus,
- Learn approaches based on recent scientific evidence,
- Examine and understand the causes of Lupus, and ultimately the best ways to treat Lupus.

This book is written in a style uniquely suited to Lupus patients, but also in a way that anyone can understand. Instead of making general statements, and leaving the patients who seek more detail at the mercy of the vague information on the Internet, I have taken a more educational and supportive approach in this text.

In the body of this text are the specific scientific and medical building blocks on which this new approach to Lupus is founded. I have decided to give the titles of key scientific articles, and the information where you can find them, right in the middle of my narrative. So, each of you and your family or friends with a scientific background can go immediately to peer-reviewed articles if you want more specific information at each point.

I am sure that you will benefit from this approach. This book explains that certain substances common in the foods Americans typically eat are responsible for triggering Lupus.

Minimizing trigger foods will improve your life!

Contents

Preface v

Introduction ix

Chapter 1: *Causes: What starts, maintains, and worsens Lupus?* 1

Chapter 2: *Mechanisms: What chemical and metabolic processes damage the body in Lupus?* 6

Chapter 3: *Treatment: Remove Lupus Triggers. Stop poisoning yourself daily* ... 12

Chapter 4: *Diagnosis: How do I know whether I really have Lupus?* 17

Chapter 5: *Medications that interfere with the guanosine pathway* 19

Chapter 6: *How reducing overall nucleotides reduces autoimmunity* 22

Chapter 7: *More on the D.A.R.T. Diet Program* 24

Chapter 8: *Prevention of the onset and progression of Lupus for women in their reproductive years* 27

Chapter 9: *Guiding principles for minimizing the lifetime risk of Lupus damage* 28

Chapter 10: *Potential Benefits of the D.A.R.T. diet for patients with other autoimmune diseases* 29

Chapter 11: *Patient Support Information* 32

Appendix I: *Primer on the immune system* 33

Appendix II: *Web portal for nucleotide content of specific foods* 38

Bibliography 39

About the Author: *Steven A. Baranowitz, MD MS MBA* 42

Introduction

This book is the culmination of more than 20 years of scientific research by dedicated physicians and scientists all over the world who have published their work in respected journals. I have used their publications as building blocks to assemble and synthesize a comprehensive understanding of Lupus and how this disease is triggered by the food we eat.

This book is organized around the most critical questions about Lupus.

Causes
What starts, maintains, and triggers worsening of Lupus?

Mechanisms
What chemical and metabolic processses act to damage my body?

Treatment
How can I remove the trigger to Lupus?

Diagnosis
How do I know whether I really have Lupus?

In my experience, most Lupus patients have tried to learn about their disease and have some familiarity with the specialized terminology of Immunology. If you don't, you may want to look at Appendix I, Primer on the Immune System, before reading the rest of this book.

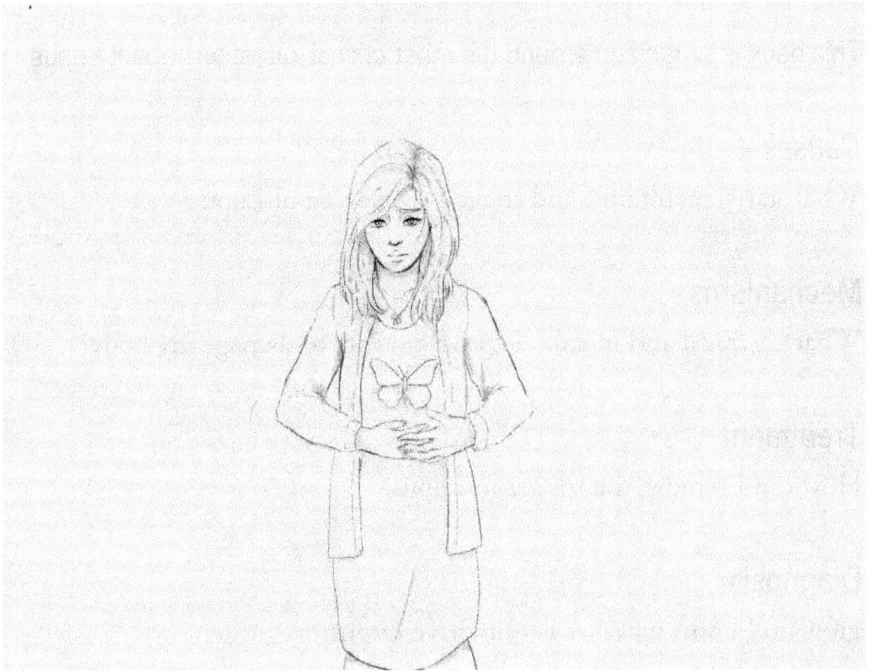

Chapter 1
Causes: What starts, maintains, and worsens Lupus?

These are the four elements that start and maintain Lupus, which is the short name for Systemic Lupus Erythematosus, or SLE.

A. The first element that triggers and maintains Lupus is production of antibodies to guanosine.

What are antibodies?

Antibodies are substances designed by our bodies to defend us against foreign invaders such as bacteria, viruses, parasites and fungi. They are produced by a special type of white blood cell called "B-lymphocytes." (See Appendix 1.) You can think of antibodies as a type of sticky glue. When they bind to an invader such as a bacterium, they produce a mass called an "immune complex."

As you know, regular glues can be specialized. For example, glass glues are different than plastic glues, which are different than metal glues.　Similarly, antibodies are specialized. Usually, each antibody has a specific target to which it attaches called an "antigen." Often antigens are proteins found on the surface of the cell.

In Lupus, instead of attaching to outside invaders, antibodies stick to parts of a person's own normal cells, causing damage and destroying those cells. The antibodies with their antigens combine to form immune complexes. The immune complex can itself do massive damage beyond that which single antibodies can do, as explained in more detail later.

What is guanosine?

Guanosine is a component of DNA, the genetic material in the nucleus of each cell. The DNA directs most of the activities of the cell and also contains all of the genetic heritage of each individual person. DNA, whose full name is "Deoxyribonucleic Acid," is made up of building blocks called nucleotides. Each nucleotide in turn contains a subunit that is called a nucleoside e.g. Guanosine, Adenosine, Thymidine and Cytidine. Nucleosides are present in all cells in the body. They are both produced and secreted by cells, and come from the breakdown of food by your digestive system.

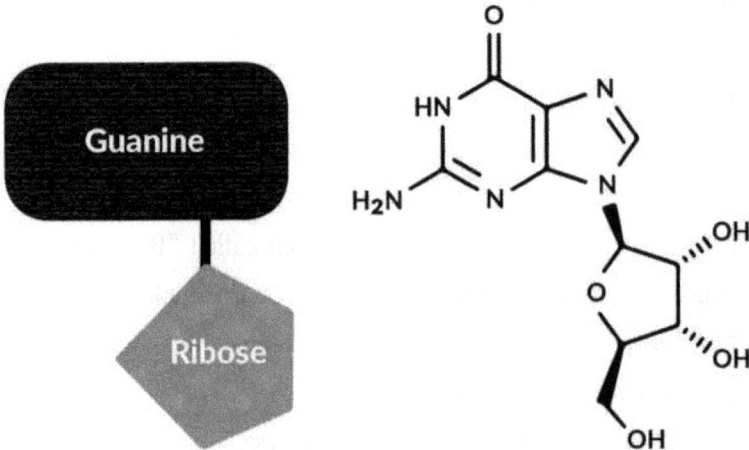

Figure 1: The icon we are using for Guanosine and its chemical structure.

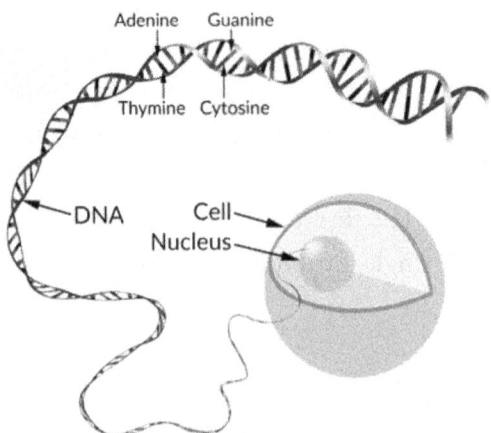

Figure 2: Guanosine contains Guanine, a component of the DNA found in the nucleus.

How does production of antibodies to guanosine cause Lupus?

People with Lupus make antibodies to many different substances. So, why are antibodies to guanosine particularly important? There are 4 main reasons:

- The presence of guanosine-containing nucleotides stimulates the production of many more antibodies than the presence of other nucleotides do.
- Combination of guanosine with "anti-guanosine antibodies" forms immune complexes which correlate with kidney damage, one of the most serious and deadly effects of Lupus.
- Anti-guanosine antibodies attach to normal cells and cause damage to several of their parts, including the mitochondria, which are the powerhouses of the cell.
- Anti-guanosine antibodies and the immune complexes can also damage the brain.

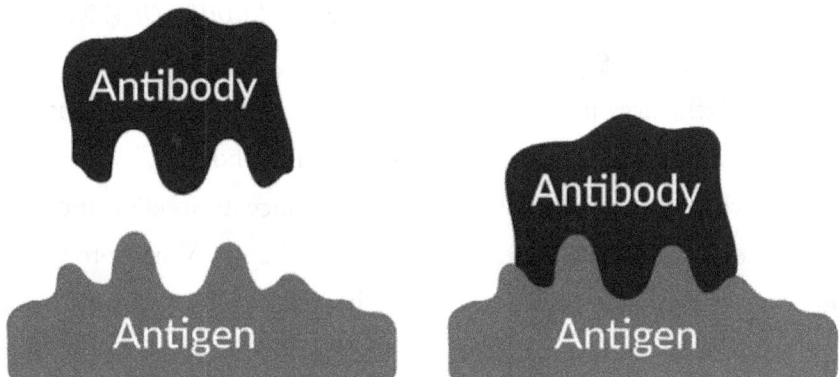

Figure 3: Formation of Antigen-Antibody Complexes

B. A second element that leads to the onset of Lupus, especially in young women, is the hormone prolactin.

Why is understanding Lupus particularly important to women?

Ninety percent of Lupus patients are women and the disease often strikes during the best times of their lives-when they have just had their first child. Understanding why women are so susceptible to Lupus, and minimizing the risk they will develop it, is critical.

What is the hormone Prolactin?

Hormones, chemical messengers produced by the body, perform many functions. Prolactin is a hormone naturally present in greater amounts in women, increasing dramatically during pregnancy, preparing breasts to produce milk for the newborn. Prolactin also has other functions.

How does Prolactin lead to the onset of Lupus for women in their reproductive years?

Prolactin influences many processes in the immune system. It interacts with the important cells we mentioned, "B-lymphocytes," which are a type of white blood cell. B-lymphocytes produce antibodies, including antibodies to guanosine, which are critical in Lupus. When prolactin is high, it results in autoimmunity-the body attacking its own cells, which is a hallmark of Lupus. Additionally, high guanosine levels in the blood seem to stimulate increased prolactin.

C. A third element is the high and unprecedented levels of guanosine in our American diet which trigger and maintain Lupus on a daily basis.

Having enough to eat was a source of great uncertainty during much of human history. Dependent on weather and farming conditions, many people ate modestly for subsistence, and famine was not uncommon. Starting with the onset of the Industrial Revolution in the late 18th and early 19th centuries, things began to change. The industrialization of agriculture has led to an unprecedented abundance, variety, and regular supply of food such as most of our ancestors never could have imagined. The epidemic of obesity, with all of its attendant diseases such as diabetes and heart attacks, that currently plagues America and most of the West, is well documented. What is not realized, is that this means that each person in the American population is taking in much more guanosine in their diet than our ancestors ever did. Most foods are rich in nucleotides, and we can roughly estimate that about a quarter of those nucleotides contain guanosine.

D. A fourth element is the misdirected and inappropriate activity of lymphocytes caused by interactions between guanosine and prolactin.

We introduced above the fact that prolactin promotes autoimmunity which is a hallmark of Lupus. Prolactin causes B-lymphocytes to misrecognize components of the body's own cells as foreign substances to be attacked. Making the situation worse is the fact that that high levels of guanosine tend to raise levels of prolactin.

Chapter 2

Mechanisms: What chemical and metabolic processes damage the body in Lupus?

1. How do antibodies to guanosine cause damage in Lupus?

Antibodies to guanosine play a critical role in the development, maintenance, and worsening of Lupus. This is an inescapable conclusion from the currently available research literature. In this chapter, I outline the key published evidence demonstrating that it is antibodies to guanosine at the core of the problem. Several published papers definitively show that both in animal models and in humans, anti-guanosine antibodies are the key. I provide short summaries of several of these papers for your review.

A ground-breaking paper in this field was published by Colburn, Green and Wong in 2001. It is entitled, "Circulating antibodies to guanosine in Systemic Lupus Erythematosus: correlation with nephritis and polyserositis by acute and longitudinal analyses." It was published in the journal *Lupus*.

Colburn and his colleagues reviewed the evidence that guanosine is the most immunogenic of the components of DNA. "Immunogenic" substances are ones that stimulate the immune system to react. They had previously conducted animal studies showing that in certain types of Lupus models, anti-guanosine antibodies proved to be the most critical. In a clinical trial they showed that the anti-guanosine antibodies correlated with the most significant symptoms and damage known to occur in people with Lupus. In fact, the anti-guanosine antibodies showed definite relationships to kidney disease, as well as with the arthritis, brain and blood problems seen in Lupus.

In a follow-up paper, Colburn and Green in 2006 extended significantly our understanding of the mechanism by which anti-guanosine antibodies cause cellular damage. It is entitled, "Serum anti-guanosine antibodies as a marker for SLE disease activity and pathogen potential," published in the journal *Clinica Chimica Acta*.

In this paper they showed that the anti-guanosine antibodies actually penetrate through the outside of the cell, then bind to mitochondria, the powerhouses of all cells, in a damaging way. The role of anti-guanosine antibodies in interfering with cell signaling, specifically involving Guanosine-binding proteins, is of enormous importance. The 2012 Nobel Prize in Chemistry was awarded to researchers who showed the indispensable role that Guanosine-binding proteins processes play in the chemistry of life. Interfering with these signaling processes clearly can contribute to the wide range of Lupus symptoms.

Other researchers have explored the interaction of anti-guanosine antibodies, and the resulting antibody-antigen immune complexes in Lupus patients, and some of those references are found at the back of this book. In addition to the direct evidence that I have just listed on how anti-guanosine antibodies cause Lupus, there are two other completely independent lines of research investigation which lead to the same conclusion.

One line concerns the sources that provide guanosine to the body. There are in fact two sources of guanosine. One is breakdown products from the food, and the other involves the synthesis of guanosine and nucleotides derived from it. The nucleotide Guanosine monophosphate, which is manufactured from guanosine, is essential for the functioning of the immune system. Regarding the synthesis of guanosine by the body itself, a drug was approved about fifteen years ago which specifically interferes with this synthetic pathway. In fact that drug, Mycophenolate, has beneficial effects on Lupus, undoubtedly because it diminishes the supply of guanosine monophosphate. The references which establish this are reviewed in chapter 5.

It has been definitively shown that reducing the overall amount of nucleotides available in the food will reduce the ability of the B-lymphocytes to proliferate and thereby manufacture antibodies. This body of evidence is reviewed in chapter 6.

2. How does the hormone Prolactin contribute to causing Lupus?

One of the more mysterious aspects of Lupus has been that 90% of those affected are women. Research has shed some light on the subject. Even a superficial review of the facts concerning prolactin and Lupus suggests a strong tie between the two. Normally women have twice as much prolactin as men, and then during pregnancy the prolactin levels increase to ten times that of their baseline. About 2% of a normal healthy population have abnormally high prolactin levels (hyperprolactinemia), whereas studies have shown that up to 33% of Lupus patients do. Good summaries of the data linking prolactin to stimulating Lupus can be found in a few recent reviews.

In 2011 Subhrajit Saha and his colleagues gave a thorough overview of the relevant data in animal models in the paper "Prolactin, Systemic Lupus Erythematosus, and Autoreactive B Cells: Lessons Learnt from Murine Models," published in the journal *Clinical Reviews in Allergy and Immunology*. In it they show in mice which naturally develop a Lupus-like syndrome, treatments which increase prolactin make Lupus worse and hasten death. They also demonstrate that in mice that normally do not develop Lupus, administration of prolactin can lead to development of a Lupus-like syndrome. This study also provides detailed information on specifically how prolactin interacts with B-lymphocytes to lead to a condition of autoimmunity in which the cells misrecognize some of the body's own cells as being foreign and therefore produce antibodies which attack them.

Then in 2012, Boaz and Orbach provide an excellent overall review of this topic called "Prolactin and Autoimmunity," published in the journal *Autoimmunity Reviews*. It gives references to the research showing the underlying mechanisms on the cellular and organismic level by which prolactin stimulates autoimmunity. It also summarizes the evidence for prolactin's involvement in autoimmunity in Lupus as well as in several other human autoimmune diseases such as Rheumatoid Arthritis and Multiple Sclerosis.

There is an important paper on the relationship between guanosine and prolactin which was published by Hill, MacLeod and Orcutt in 1976 in the journal *Endocrinology* titled "Dibutyryl cyclic AMP, adenosine and guanosine blockade of the dopamine, ergocryptine and apomorphine inhibition of prolactin release in vitro." They showed in an animal model that guanosine increased prolactin. This raises the distinct possibility that increased guanosine exposure in humans also leads to increased levels of prolactin and thus the autoimmunity which characterizes Lupus. It is clear that the hormone prolactin can contribute to bringing about and/or worsening Lupus, and likely that high levels of guanosine increase the amount of prolactin in the body.

3. How do high and unprecedented levels of guanosine in our American diet trigger and maintain Lupus on a daily basis?

Today, and more so than ever in our history, obesity is epidemic, and for many Americans there is food lurking everywhere to tempt them all the time.

A government report indicated that Americans in the late 20th century took in about 2000 mg of nucleotides in their diet on an average day. If we roughly estimate that a quarter of these contain guanosine, then we have roughly 500 mg of guanosine per day in the diet. Our bodies also manufacture guanosine from precursor molecules, and further assemble it into nucleotides such as guanosine monophosphate.

It is common knowledge that the variety and abundance of food in the mid to late twentieth century and beyond is greater for Americans than ever in our history. And since nucleotides are present in virtually every meal, so is the amount of guanosine-containing nucleotides.

However, the human race, which evolved over many tens of thousands of years, developed bodies which were typically exposed to limited amounts and less variety of food during all of that time, except for the last approximately 70-100 years of our existence. Therefore they were exposed to less guanosine, whereas now we are clearly exposed to unprecedented amounts of guanosine on a daily basis. In this situation, instead of getting just enough guanosine to subsist, we are now exposed to an excess amount that is acting like an injected drug. It is this oversupply which is responsible for the autoimmunity that is characteristic of Lupus.

As mentioned above, in addition to the guanosine we take in through the diet, our bodies also manufacture guanosine. The view that excess guanosine is harmful is further reinforced by data from the drug mycophenolate, which interferes with guanosine monophosphate synthesis in the body thus lowering the overall body exposure to guanosine. Mycophenolate clearly improves many patients with Lupus in this way.

4. How is the misdirected and inappropriate activity of lymphocytes caused by interactions of guanosine and prolactin?

An enormous amount of research has been published which focuses on the details of how lymphocytes misbehave and cause damage in Lupus. Like many investigations in biology, it has been hard to determine what is cause and what is effect regarding these aberrant lymphocyte actions.

Because there is such a wide variety of different antibodies made by Lupus patients, it has been very difficult to ascertain which ones seem to be critical to causing the disease. However, the data laid out above supports the conclusion that guanosine and prolactin and their interaction in fact are the key factors ultimately causing the onset, maintenance, and worsening of Lupus in most patients. Naturally some individuals are more genetically susceptible than others.

The following are some of the abnormal behavior of lymphocytes documented in Lupus, and as a result of excess guanosine and high levels of prolactin:

- B-lymphocytes make anti-guanosine antibodies which do a great deal of body damage.
- B-lymphocytes make a wide range of other antibodies which do varying degrees of damage.
- Autoimmunity is promoted by the way prolactin interacts with
  - B-lymphocytes.
- T-lymphocytes also become abnormal.

Chapter 3 - Treatment

Remove Lupus Triggers. Stop poisoning yourself daily

Summary of rationale for low-guanosine diet in Lupus patients.

The Common Sense Approach

How reducing the amount of guanosine in your diet will improve your symptoms and mitigate the disease.

All of the information and experimental data reviewed in the preceding chapters leads to one clear conclusion - excess guanosine in the American diet both causes and aggravates the symptoms of Lupus. So let's think about treating Lupus in a similar way to how other food-related diseases are treated.

For instance, if you are allergic to strawberries and they give you hives, the treatment is pretty simple: Don't eat strawberries! If you are diabetic, and too much sugar can act as a poison which can put you in to coma or kill you, every diabetic knows how to act: Carefully limit the amount of sugar in your food! And similarly, for Lupus patients whose disease is initiated and made worse by excess guanosine in their foods, it is only common sense that they need to limit their intake of guanosine.

How reducing the amount of nucleotides in your diet will tamp down the extreme and misdirected activity of your lymphocytes.

Reducing guanosine intake will immediately have two favorable effects on Lupus and specifically B-lymphocytes.

First, if there is less guanosine in the body, then the B-lymphocytes will be less stimulated to make anti-guanosine antibodies.

As we discussed in the opening chapters, it is these antibodies that are directly responsible for much of the damage that Lupus does.

Second, if there is less of the nucleotide guanosine monophosphate taken in to the body, then the B-lymphocytes will be less able to multiply (as discussed in chapter 5) and therefore less able to produce anti-guanosine antibodies.

The D.A.R.T. Diet

Dietary Autoimmunity Reduction Therapy

1. How the diet was formulated

If you look on the box for any food in the US, you will see listings of several of its contents, including protein, fats, carbohydrates, sodium, and others. One thing it is unlikely you will ever see is a listing of the nucleic acids such as guanosine or adenosine. Yet most types of food contains nucleic acids, and specifically the amount of guanosine is critical to patients who have Lupus.

In order to design specialized diets that are low in guanosine, I was pleased to have the consulting services of an excellent research dietitian, Sara Schaeffer, M.A., R.D., L.D.N. Together, we extensively reviewed all sources worldwide that we could obtain concerning the nucleotide content of foods, including scientific publications in foreign languages that needed to be translated and various databases. It was surprising that there was rather little in the US research literature on this topic and that most of what existed was European. The information we uncovered was enough to construct diets that would meaningfully reduce the daily intake of guanosine, and yet be balanced in all other respects and be tasty.

Methods of food preparation and the diversity of food Americans eat have changed considerably over the last 50 years, so we also identified an ongoing need for new research in terms of the nucleic acid components of US foods. We are currently putting together research planning to update the information available with new research measurements and technologies. But for now, the diets we have constructed will be entirely adequate to assist Lupus patients in minimizing their disease.

2. How it works as a type of nutrition therapy, not a weight loss diet.

Management of your diet to improve Lupus is directed at attacking your disease and prolonging your life. You can't cheat on your diet and expect that your body won't notice!

Your body is exquisitely and unfortunately sensitive to every guanosine molecule that you take in and to the overall amounts of nucleotides that you consume every day. The dietary management of Lupus is not something that is directed to helping you lose weight, and a little food cheating can wipe out weeks of careful attention to diet. Although it is possible that you may lose weight while on this diet as a beneficial side effect, the diet is constructed so that you have all of the normal required and balanced nutrients that your body needs.

3. The variations in the diet and how they are applied.

In designing the diet, one of the guiding principles is that a "one size fits all" diet would not be medically appropriate. This is true in other food sensitive diseases such as diabetes or kidney insufficiency. The diet must be individually appropriate to each person's particular medical situation.

We created a system of reference tiers for diets:

- Most Restrictive (lowest nucleotide content; for emergencies.)

- Standard Restrictive diet
- Modestly Restrictive
- Maintenance

4. Key components of the D.A.R.T. program.

The diet program is comprised of an initial period of about 6 months, during which the physician and dietician evaluate and work to optimize diet treatment for each Lupus patient. The physician initially evaluates the severity of the patient's disease based on signs and symptoms, laboratory tests, evidence of organ damage, etc, and then recommends a specific diet. The patient is followed over the next few months with repeat followup disease evaluations and diet adjustments by the physician. The patient may be asked to keep, as individually necessary, diaries of symptoms such as headaches, skin rashes, joint pains, etc. These diaries are periodically reviewed by the physician.

The dietician has an initial meeting with the patient in which the practical aspects of the diet program are explained in detail. This first visit includes describing weighing the foods to be included in the diet, characterizing the portion size for each type of food, keeping a food diary, advising on the effect of cooking on food nucleotide content, etc. The patient will have one or more followup visits, as well as occasional phone, email or other communications with the dietician to answer questions and direct the treatment.

Depending on the severity of the patient's disease, an initial diet will be selected. As the patient stabilizes clinically or based on laboratory testing, the patient will be moved through a series of diets with increasing nucleotide content but which are still substantially low compared to the typical Western diet. It is believed that for each patient there is a threshold for reactivity, and that if the diets are below that threshold the patient will have successfully minimized signs, symptoms, and progression of Lupus. The goal of the program is then to put the patient on a convenient and palatable maintenance diet which they can follow for a period of years.

It is important to note that at least in the first six months patients remain on whatever prescription medications they are currently taking. Usually prescription medications such as chloroquine or immunosuppressives are managed by the patient's physician. It is expected that when the patient's blood tests, signs and symptoms improve during the course of the diet, the physician may well decide to lower or discontinue some of these prescription medications.

In this way patients need not worry that the dietary therapy may require any changes in medications they are currently on, especially if those medications seem to be keeping them stable.

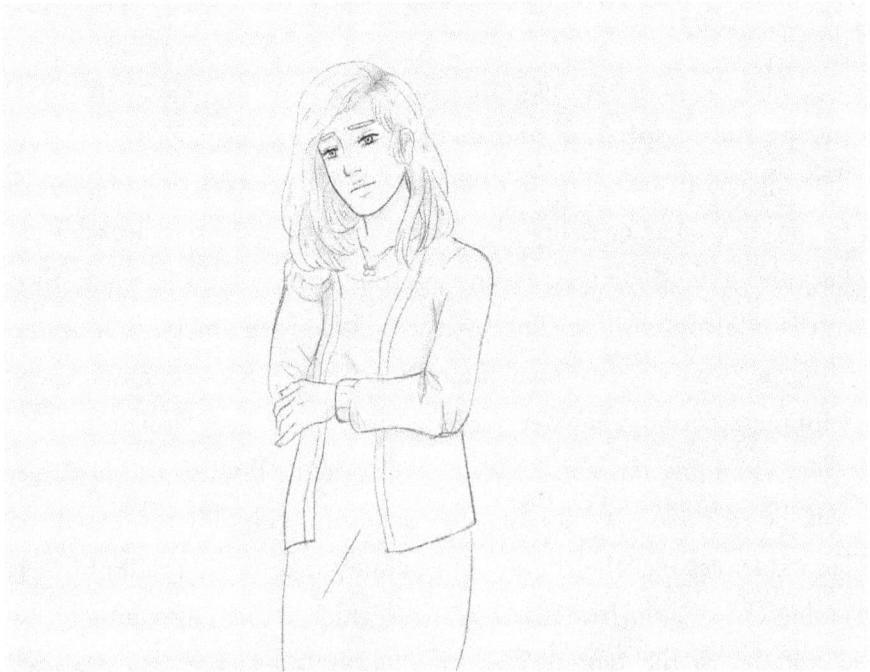

Chapter 4
Diagnosis: How do I know whether I really have Lupus?

If you are reading this book, it is likely that your doctor has told you that you have Lupus, or that you have a loved one who has been told that they have Lupus. Most of the time, the doctor will have been correct in his diagnosis, but the diagnosis of Lupus has always been and remains fundamentally a clinical diagnosis - in other words it is dependent on a physician's judgment. There is no one single blood test historically which alone will permit the unequivocal diagnosis of Lupus. There are many different signs, symptoms and evaluation of different organs that are affected by Lupus. Because diagnosis is so complex, it is usually best managed by a rheumatologist and/or a dermatologist who has a lot of training and practical experience in the whole range of autoimmune diseases.

General medical doctors including primary care, internal medicine, family practice, and even gynecologists, pediatricians, and others can be good at picking up symptoms suggestive of autoimmune diseases, but it is best to have the patient subsequently evaluated by a specialist such as a rheumatologist and/or a dermatologist.

Lupus in some cases may overlap with other autoimmune diseases and the precise diagnosis in these cases may involve a substantial number of blood tests and other diagnostic tests to sort out. Some autoimmune diseases have symptoms which are similar, and some patients have more than one autoimmune disease. In fact, Lupus has been called "the great imitator" because of this difficulty to diagnose. The symptoms of Lupus are many times indistinguishable from symptoms of rheumatoid arthritis, blood disorders, fibromyalgia, diabetes, thyroid problems, Lyme disease, and other various heart, lung, muscle, and bone diseases.

Because Lupus affects your entire body, a wide range of symptoms is known to occur. Some symptoms will come and go, disappearing and reappearing at different times during the course of the disease, further confusing diagnosis. Common symptoms of Lupus include:

- Butterfly-shaped rash (on cheeks and nose)
- Light-sensitivity
- Hair loss
- Fingers turning white and/or blue in cold
- Headaches
- Painful and swollen joints

One of the more pernicious aspects of Lupus is that sometimes it will start in a single organ and then will be misdiagnosed as a primary disease of that organ. For instance in some people Lupus seems to manifest first in the brain and they may be misdiagnosed as having a psychiatric disorder for years, when instead it is due to Lupus. Similarly, in some cases Lupus first manifests in the kidney and then it may be misdiagnosed as a primary kidney disease.

It is my hope that as research on Lupus progresses, a definitive single blood test will become available which will be the standard for its diagnosis.

Chapter 5
Medications that interfere with the guanosine pathway

The fact that guanosine is a critical element in the immune system has been known for about two decades to physicians involved in transplantation of organs. The drug mycophenolate works by restricting a derivative of guanosine, guanosine monophosphate, from being produced by the body. This in turn limits the ability of lymphocytes to proliferate, meaning that the production of antibodies by B-lymphocytes and related functions performed by T-lymphocytes are reduced. The drug is effective in suppressing the immune system during transplantation. In fact, mycophenolate is beneficial for many patients with Lupus and continues to be used.

One of the rather peculiar facts about the research literature concerning mycophenolate is that there is very little mention of the fact that guanosine monophosphate and other forms of guanosine are available to the body from the foods we ingest.

Not recognizing the importance of diet as a source of guanosine and its derivatives has two rather surprising results. First, doctors who prescribe mycophenolate do not recommend that the patients restrict their food intake amounts of guanosine and guanosine monophosphate. Nowhere in the FDA official approved labeling (package insert) are there any recommendations to do so. So while the drug works hard to reduce the body's production of guanosine monophosphate to reduce the activity of the immune system, patients are still taking in large amounts of guanosine, which reduces the effectiveness of the drug. This may also contribute to the variability in the effectiveness of the drug in different patients, as the amount of guanosine monophosphate in the diet will vary. Second, neither doctors nor patients have understood that they may be able to achieve similar results to what is seen with the drug mycophenolate, or perhaps better results, simply by restricting guanosine intake. In the next chapter we review information assembled in the last few decades by other research groups that restricting the nucleotide content of foods can have a dramatic result in reducing activity of the immune system.

Therefore, the concept that patients with Lupus should be on diets which are low in guanosine and its derivatives has the potential to benefit patients in many different ways. If they are able to achieve results in reducing Lupus signs and symptoms which are as good or better than that of the prescription drug mycophenolate, then they will be able to discontinue the mycophenolate, avoiding side effects which mycophenolate carries with it. If patients using mycophenolate also have guanosine reduced diets when they are taking the drug, then it is likely the drug will be more effective and deliver more consistent results. Since mycophenolate is useful in other diseases, the adoption of dietary restriction at the same time the drug is used may also benefit patients with these other diseases.

There are numerous published studies showing that mycophenolate is beneficial to patients with Lupus. Conti and colleagues in 2014 published the study, "Mycophenolate mofetil in systemic Lupus erythematosus: results from a retrospective study in a large monocentric cohort and review of the literature" in the journal *Immunological Research*. They evaluated over 600 patients with Lupus, closely following their progress. After only four months there was significant, measurable, and objective improvement due to use of mycophenolate. Patients with and without kidney disease benefited.

In 2011, Maria Dall'Era and her colleagues published "Mycophenolate mofetil in the treatment of systemic Lupus erythematosus" in *Current Opinion in Rheumatology*. The purpose of this paper was to review evidence from recent large studies concerning use of mycophenolate for Lupus, especially in comparison to other immunosuppressives such as azathioprine. It concluded that 10 years of clinical trials clearly demonstrate that mycophenolate benefits patients with Lupus.

Chapter 6
*How reducing overall nucleotides
reduces autoimmunity*

There is an extensive body of literature which definitively establishes that reducing the nucleotide content of foods can reduce the responsiveness of the immune system. I have been surprised that apparently no one, as far as I can tell, has published information indicating that they have systematically tried to create diets which are low in nucleotides to apply them as medical nutrition therapy. There are numerous studies which suggest this would be of enormous benefit to patients with Lupus as well as other autoimmune diseases.

The general importance of nucleotides in human foods is well-established. A good place to start reading about the basic information available on this topic, especially for readers with a background in college science or nutrition, would be the publication by Carver and Walker, entitled "The role of nucleotides in human nutrition," published in the journal *Nutritional Biochemistry*.

Then to narrow our focus from the many general metabolism functions in which nucleotides are involved, to their role in the immune system, we can utilize the excellent review by Kulkarni, Rudolph and Van Buren, entitled, "Dietary sources of nucleotides in immune function: a review," published in the journal *Nutrition* in 1994. This article concisely summarizes the history of discovery that nucleotides from food not only participate in the immune system, but also regulate some of its key processes. It also goes over several key studies showing that reduction of nucleotides in the diet can reduce undesirable overactivity of the immune system.

As we have discussed, Lupus is a disease in which there is massive overactivity of the immune system toward the body's own components, and this involves classically a tremendous overproduction of antibodies by B-lymphocytes. There are quite a few publications that discuss the influence of nucleotides on the secretion of antibodies by B-lymphocytes. One interesting paper is that by Navarro and his colleagues entitled "Modulation of antibody forming cell and mitogen driven lymphoproliferative responses by dietary nucleotides in mice," and this was published in the journal *Immunology Letters*. This paper shows in a mouse model that guanosine monophosphate increases the amount of antibodies which are produced. Of course this is undesirable in Lupus which classically has been understood as a disease of oversupply of antibodies that would attach to one's own cells.

The papers just mentioned are just the tip of the iceberg in terms of the substantial literature showing that restriction of dietary nucleotides can reduce an overactive immune system's destructive activities. It seems only common sense that reducing the dietary intake of guanosine and related substances in the diet of Lupus patients is just as important to their health as is reducing the sugar intake in patients who have diabetes.

Chapter 7
More on the D.A.R.T. Diet Program

Each Lupus patient is unique.

The signs, symptoms, and medical history of every patient with Lupus tends to be more variable than we often see in other diseases. However they are consistent with the wide range of clinical conditions which characterize other autoimmune diseases.

This clinical variability has confused generations of physicians and investigators and led to uncountable attempts to reclassify and subclassify the different types of Lupus so as to understand its essence and improve its diagnosis and treatment. The concepts that I have put forward in this book, and especially the primacy of guanosine and prolactin in starting, maintaining, and worsening of Lupus, make possible a new approach to treatment.

The best way to treat any disease is simply to remove the cause of the disease, rather than to try to treat the myriad signs, symptoms and complications. The Dietary Autoimmunity Reduction Therapy program is therefore the first step in this new approach.

Patients with Lupus range from those to whom it is a minor inconvenience to those whom it is bringing to death's door. Patients vary in how old they were when they were diagnosed with the disease, how many years they have had it, whether they have kidney, brain, skin or other severe organ involvement, what prescription medications they are on, and what side effects to these medications they encounter, etc.

We are starting to accept patients for treatment into the D.A.R.T. program. Each one will have the personalized individual evaluation by a physician that each Lupus patient requires. They will then be classified to a particular reference tier diet, and then that diet will be further individualized for each patient during the course of treatment by weekly analysis of their diet and by their objective responses. This is done by the physician and the Lupus nutritionist in the program.

Patients will all need to keep a detailed diary of their meals, and how many servings of each food they have, and the nucleotide intake of each individual patient is then calculated every week. Patients with a history of headaches, which are common among Lupus patients, will also keep a headache diary to assess their progress.

Currently, I estimate that for many Lupus patients it will take about three months of the diet for them to show a clear response in reducing their signs and symptoms. Three months is not a long time for improvement if you consider that many have had their disease for years and in some measure will suffer from it for their entire lifetimes (despite current conventional treatment).

Once clear improvement is demonstrated, patients will have to remain on the diet they are on for another few months to stabilize their condition. After that, I believe they will be able to move to a maintenance diet less restrictive than the one they have initially been treated with. The maintenance diet will be easier for them to follow in the future so as to continue to keep their Lupus under control.

Papers published by Colburn's group indicate that anti-guanosine antibody blood tests would be the most effective way of monitoring the process of the diet. However, at the time of writing of this book such tests are not commercially available, and they are only research laboratory tests. One test that is commercially available is the double-stranded DNA test, which although not as precise as the anti- guanosine antibody test, does give a pretty good measure of disease activity, and is much better than the more common Anti-Nuclear Antibody blood test. So I use the dsDNA test to monitor the patients progress, along with evaluating other signs and symptoms of the disease.

At the beginning of the dietary treatment program and at least for several months afterwards, patients will generally stay on whatever prescription medicines they have been on. Only when they show objective improvement in their signs, symptoms and other tests of their functions are prescription medications diminished or discontinued. Also, when patients have flares (worsening) of their Lupus, they need to be rapidly and effectively treated by the physician with prescription medications, and then afterward appropriately tapered off most prescription medications as soon as their condition will allow.

It is important to understand that this nutrition modification therapy is fundamentally different than a weight-loss type diet. Management of your food intake of nucleotides to improve Lupus is directed at attacking your disease and prolonging your life.

I repeat the information mentioned above because it is so important: You can't cheat on your diet and expect that your body won't notice! Your body is exquisitely and unfortunately sensitive to every guanosine molecule that you take in and to the overall amounts of nucleotides that you consume every day. Once again, the dietary management of Lupus is not something that is directed to helping you lose weight, and a little food cheating can wipe out weeks of careful attention to diet. Although it is possible that you may lose weight while on this diet as a beneficial side effect, the diet is constructed so that you have all of the normal required and balanced nutrients that your body requires.

Chapter 8

Prevention of the onset and progression of Lupus
for women in their reproductive years

Women in their childbearing years, menarche to menopause, as a result of this book, need to have a recognition of the role that guanosine-containing nucleotides (and other nucleotides) in the diet can play in triggering Lupus. While some degree of nucleotides in the diet is normal and indispensable, the extreme levels present in the typical American diet currently can be dangerous and trigger Lupus.

Women who are pregnant or planning to become pregnant need to be especially careful in their diet, because the increase in prolactin in their bodies during pregnancy and the potential interaction of guanosine in the diet to increase the levels of prolactin will likely predispose them to developing Lupus.

Patients who start to take certain medications known to cause Lupus, e.g. procainamide, should be careful to minimize the amount of nucleotides in their diet. If possible, they should do this for several weeks before they start the medication, and report to their physician any Lupus like symptoms immediately

People who have relatives with Lupus may have a genetic predisposition to it. They should be careful to follow diets with a reduced amount of guanosine-containing, and other nucleotides, to help prevent Lupus. Also, they should be tested yearly for Lupus by the anti-dsDNA test or more specific tests for anti-guanosine antibodies, if these become commonly available.

Chapter 9

Guiding principles for minimizing the lifetime risk of Lupus damage

Because the course of Lupus over a lifetime has been historically unpredictable, is important for patients to do whatever they can to minimize progression of this potentially fatal disease.

Here are some of the key steps needed to take in this regard.

1. If you ever have had a single positive ANA blood test, you should be checked yearly with a repeat of this test and of the double-stranded DNA test, whether or not you have additional or new signs and symptoms. Lupus can develop many years after an initial positive ANA test and it can develop very suddenly. It is best to diagnose it as early as possible.

2. If you have been diagnosed by only a general medical doctor, you should then be evaluated by a rheumatologist or a dermatologist to confirm the diagnosis by a specialist.

3. Patients who wish to be evaluated for treatment in the D.A.R.T. diet program should contact our office by using the contact form on our website or by calling our office number.

4. Patients with Lupus need to minimize their exposure to the sun and minimize their exposure to cold.

5. Whenever patients see new specialists, or are hospitalized for any reason, they should tell their doctors that they have been diagnosed with Lupus, and should always have a copy of their most recent blood tests.

6. Patients who have kidney disease need to be followed by a nephrologist (kidney specialist)

Chapter 10
Potential Benefits of the D.A.R.T. diet for patients with other autoimmune diseases

It is likely that the high levels of guanosine-containing nucleotides (and other nucleotides) in the typical American diet predispose us to other widespread diseases. These include many autoimmune diseases, as well as some diseases that are generally considered idiopathic (the cause is not known), such as essential hypertension and Type II diabetes.

In any case, it seems that reduction of the guanosine and its derivatives in the body is a good thing in many diseases. In fact, mycophenolate, which as discussed above is a prescription drug which reduces the body content of guanosine monophosphate, has shown effectiveness in a wide range of diseases, including diseases such as systemic sclerosis, essential hypertension, fibrosis, and others. It would seem clear that the D.A.R.T. diet has the potential to benefit patients in all those diseases where mycophenolate has shown effectiveness. Logically, because the D.A.R.T. diet reduces guanosine monophosphate and thereby reduces proliferation of both B cells and T cells, it is expected that it will be able to make a significant difference for patients with a broad variety of autoimmune diseases.

The following is a list of some of the autoimmune diseases which have been shown to respond to mycophenolate, and which therefore would be expected to benefit from the D.A.R.T. diet program. Mycophenolate was shown to be effective in published human studies for most of these diseases, but in some the data come from animal models of human diseases. Although one reference is listed for each disease, often there are multiple published papers available on each disease.

Autoimmune Hepatitis. Sharzehi, K. *et al.* 2010. Mycophenolate mofetil for the treatment of autoimmune hepatitis in patients refractory or intolerant to conventional therapy. *Can J Gastroenterol* 24: 588-592.

Autoimmune Inflammatory Myopathy. Majithia, V. *et al.* 2005. Mycophenolate mofetil (CellCept): an alternative therapy for autoimmune inflammatory myopathy. *Rheumatology (Oxford)* 44: 386-389.

Dermatomyositis. Rouster-Stevens, K. A. *et al.* 2010. Mycophenolate mofetil: a possible therapeutic agent for children with juvenile dermatomyositis. *Arthritis Care Res (Hoboken)* 62: 1446-1451.

Diabetes. Ugrasbul, F. *et al.* 2008. Prevention of diabetes: effect of mycophenolate mofetil and anti-CD25 on onset of diabetes in the DRBB rat. *Pediatr Diabetes* 9: 596-601.

Graft Versus Host Disease. Furlong, T. *et al.* 2009. Therapy with mycophenolate mofetil for refractory acute and chronic GVHD. *Bone Marrow Transplant* 44: 739-748.

Idiopathic Thrombocytopenic Purpura. Zhang, W. *et al.* 2005. Mycophenolate mofetil as a treatment for refractory idiopathic thrombocytopenic purpura. *Acta Pharmacol Sin* 26: 598-602.

Myositis. Pisoni, C. *et al.* 2007. Mycophenolate mofetil treatment in resistant myositis. *Rheumatology (Oxford)* 46: 516-518.

Pemphigus vulgaris. Koga, H., *et al.* 2010. Successful treatment with mycophenolate mofetil of four Japanese patients with pemphigus vulgaris. *Eur J Dermatol* 20: 472-475.

Pyoderma Grangrenosum. Lee, M *et al.* 2004. Mycophenolate mofetil in pyoderma gangrenosum. *J Dermatolog Treat* 15: 303-307.

Sarcoid. O'Connor, A.S. *et al.* 2003. Pancreatitis and duodenitis from sarcoidosis: successful therapy with mycophenolate mofetil. *Dig Dis Sci* 48: 2191-2195.

Systemic Sclerosis (Scleroderma). Nihtyanova, S.I. *et al.* 2007 Mycophenolate mofetil in diffuse cutaneous systemic sclerosis—a retrospective analysis. *Rheumatology (Oxford)*. 46:442-5.

Uveitis. Daniel, E., *et al.* 2010. Mycophenolate mofetil for ocular inflammation. *Am J Ophthalmol* 149: 423-32.

Vasculitis. Nikibakhsh, A.A., *et al.* 2010. Treatment of complicated Henoch-Schönlein Purpura with mycophenolate mofetil: a retrospective case series report. *Int J Rheumatol* 2010: 254316, doi:10.1155/2010/254316.

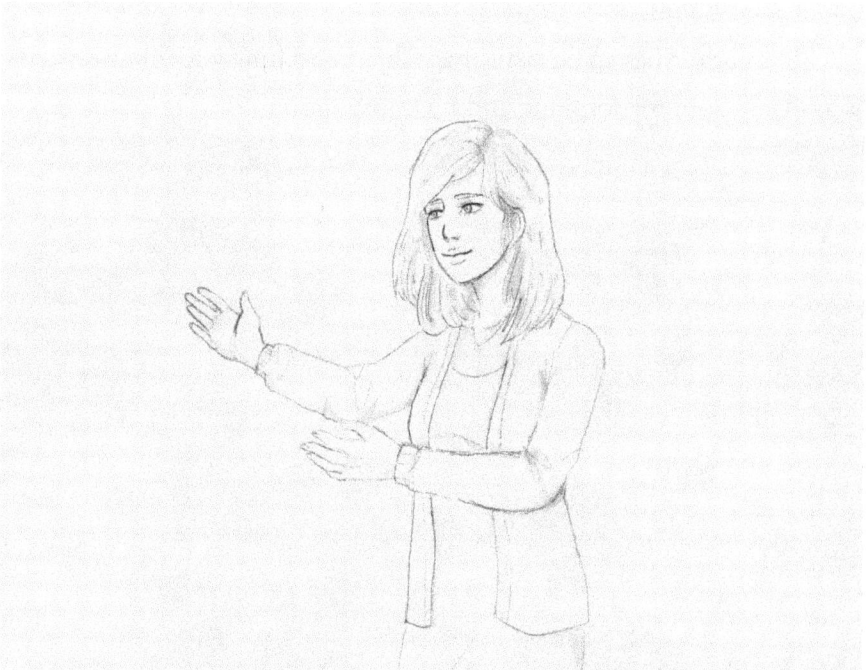

Chapter 11
Patient Support Information

Patients who wish to be evaluated for Dietary Autoimmunity Reduction Therapy should contact us by our website or calling our office.

For those who wish to know the relative nucleotide content of specific foods, we will be enabling them to access our database and submit specific foods that they wish to find out about.

The bibliography lists extensive articles about Lupus, most of which can be obtained from a university library, or from your local library by interlibrary loan. The core concepts of many of these articles will be especially helpful to anyone who has taken some college level biology classes, or who is willing to read an introductory textbook on immunology. In Appendix I of this book, we provide a very simplified introduction to the basic knowledge of immunology needed to understand Lupus.

The author has spoken on this subject to Lupus organizations, and is available both for speaking and for consultations.

Appendix I

Primer on the immune system

A. Introduction to basic immunology

It's a jungle out there! Although we don't normally think of it day to day, our bodies are coated with lots of microorganisms, such as bacteria, viruses and fungi. They all live normally in our skin and on our hair, as well as internally in our stomachs, and our intestines. We normally don't think about the fact that our bodies are continuously under attack from all types of microorganisms.

We have the luxury of not worrying about these things usually, because we have an automatic defense system which is supremely effective most of the time in defending us from all attacks. This is the immune system. It has its shock troops, its foot soldiers, it's command-and-control, its sophisticated networks of communication systems, which most of the time work flawlessly to keep out invaders.

In this brief Appendix, I will give a basic outline of the way the immune system is structured. I will focus on the cells (see Fig. 4) that comprise the immune system, because that is the information most immediately relevant to understanding Lupus. The embryology and evolution of the immune system, the anatomy of the different organs, the cell signaling network, and other fascinating aspects will not be dealt with in this brief section.

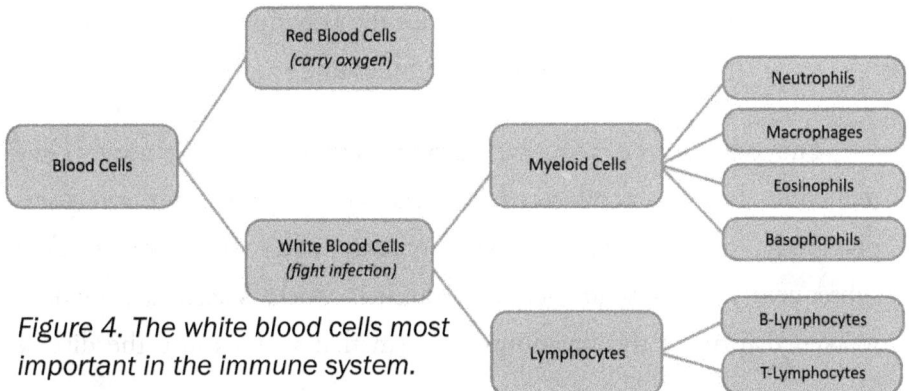

Figure 4. The white blood cells most important in the immune system.

Often it is useful to subclassify the immune system cells into comprising the Innate system, which is the oldest evolutionarily, and the Adaptive system, which is newer.

The cells in the Innate immune system include:
- Macrophages - Engulf and destroy bacteria.
- Neutrophils - Release chemicals to demolish invading organisms.
- Basophils - Secrete chemicals which damage invading organisms.
- Eosinophils - Fight parasites and are involved in certain types of allergic reactions.
- Mast Cells - Mainly concerned with allergic response.

The cells in the Adaptive immune system include:
- B-lymphocytes - Factories for antibodies, which are molecules found in the blood that attach to foreign substances to inactivate and destroy them. They provide "humoral immunity."
- T-lymphocytes - These engage in what is called "cell-mediated immunity." In a variety of ways, they approach the dangerous invading microorganisms and neutralize them. There are many subtypes of T-lymphocytes, and some of these cooperate with the B-lymphocytes so as to help the B-lymphocytes to function.

The cells of the adaptive immune system have memory. They remember having encountered bacteria, viruses and other foreigners previously, and can respond very quickly when they are attacked subsequently. This is in fact how vaccines work. Vaccines provide a weakened form of the invading organism that won't cause the disease but teach the immune system how to recognize them early nonetheless. Lymphocytes are critically dependent for their functions on guanosine monophosphate, which is depicted in Fig. 5 below.

Many cell types cooperate in various ways with each other during invasion by bacteria or viruses. For example, macrophages act as "antigen-presenting cells" to lymphocytes, providing them with information to help the lymphocytes target the invaders.

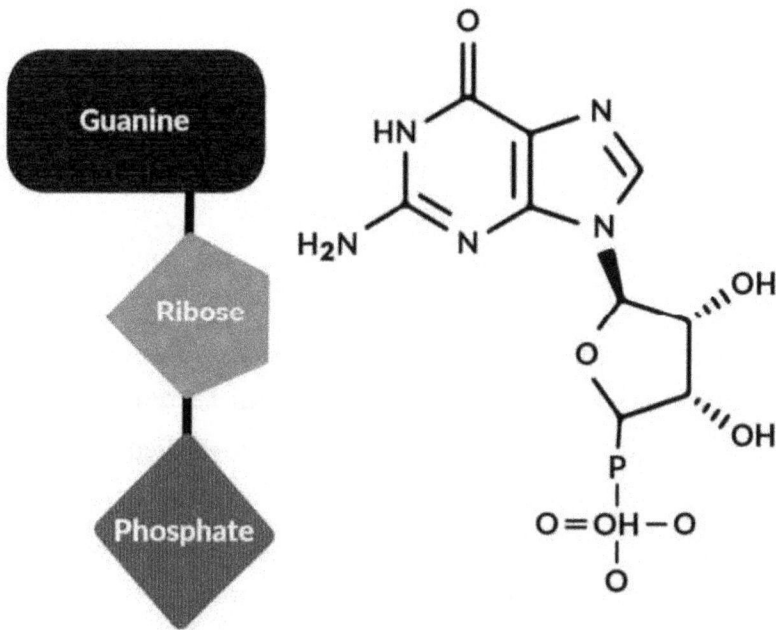

Figure 5. Guanosine Monophosphate Icon and Chemical structure

B. The fundamentals of Lupus autoimmunity

Lupus is one form of what are called "autoimmune diseases," in which our immune system malfunctions and attack the normal cells of our own bodies. Other examples are Rheumatoid Arthritis and Crohn's Disease, but there are many others. Studied by many hundreds of researchers over the last 70 years, most of this research has centered on identifying abnormalities in the functioning of the immune system, in the hope of identifying key factors which cause and exacerbate the disease.

What is classically taught about Lupus reflects the condition which is seen in many areas of science when researchers are only at the stage of collecting large amounts of information, but have no general organizing principles for this data. To get a general idea of the massive amount of data which has been accumulated about the immune system in Lupus, you might want to consult a textbook, such as *Systemic Lupus Erythematosus* edited by Robert G. Lahita. This book has hundreds of pages which deal with just summarizing some of the immunology research on Lupus.

The information below only provides the simplest entry to understanding the available information on the autoimmunity which is the hallmark of Lupus. One of the earliest and most enduring pieces of evidence indicating that Lupus involved the immune system attacking a person's own cells, was provided by the Anti-Nuclear Antibody test, which is still widely used today. Essentially, it demonstrated that factors were being produced that attacked the nuclei of their own cells. These factors are antibodies. However, in Lupus patients, antibodies interact not only with the nuclei of cells, but with many other parts of the cell. In fact, over a hundred types of antibodies have identified. See the 2014 report by Yaniv and colleagues - "Volcanic explosion of autoantibodies in systemic Lupus erythematosus: A diversity of 180 different antibodies found in SLE patients." in *Autoimmun Rev*.

Researchers have spent a lot of time cataloging all these antibodies and trying to figure out what are the potential causes and effects of all of their actions. They have tried to understand the mechanisms by which immune cells are stimulated to produce such antibodies, and how the antibodies cause the organ damage. Only in the last 20 years have researchers also realized the hormone prolactin along with other hormones contribute substantially to creating conditions where people are inclined to develop antibodies against the body's own cells. In fact, although historically prolactin has been understood as being produced in the pituitary gland, it is also produced in important immune cells such as lymphocytes and macrophages.

This brief introduction to Lupus autoimmunity may help patients with little exposure to the concepts of the immune system to understand, as they read the chapters in this book, how Lupus is triggered, maintained, and worsened by guanosine exposure in susceptible individuals.

Appendix II
Web portal for nucleotide content of specific foods

Lupus patients reading this book will naturally be curious as to how foods they regularly eat measure up in terms of their content of damage-causing guanosine.

As a tool for patients use in answering that question, we will be making available a website which provides information on the relative content of guanosine in different foods from our proprietary database. Patients can search the database for the guanosine content of some of their typical foods.

We emphasize that as of today, only the physician and dietician managed D.A.R.T. diet program, represents a sound comprehensive approach to reducing the foods which trigger Lupus, while maintaining good nutrition overall. Interested patients should make an appointment for a personal medical evaluation.

Bibliography

Carver, J.D. and Walker, W.A. 1995. The role of nucleotides in human nutrition. *Nutritional Biochemistry* 6: 58-72.

Colburn, K.K. and Green, L.M. Serum anti-guanosine antibodies as a marker for SLE disease activity and pathogen potential. *Clinica Chimica Acta*, 370: 9-16.

Colburn, K.K., Green, L.M. and Wong, A.K. 2001. Circulating antibodies to guanosine in Systemic Lupus Erythematosus: correlation with nephritis and polyserositis by acute and longitudinal analyses. *Lupus*, 10:410-417.

Conti, F., *et al.*, 2014. Mycophenolate mofetil in Systemic Lupus Erythematosus: results from a retrospective study in a large monocentric cohort and review of the literature. *Immunological Research* 60: 270-276.

Dall'Era, M. 2011. Mycophenolate mofetil in the treatment of Systemic Lupus Erythematosus. *Curr Opin Rheumatol* 23: 454-8.

Daniel, E., *et al.* 2010. Mycophenolate mofetil for ocular inflammation. *Am J Ophthalmol* 149: 423-32.

Furlong, T. *et al.* 2009. Therapy with mycophenolate mofetil for refractory acute and chronic GVHD. *Bone Marrow Transplant* 44: 739-748.

Hill, M.K., MacLeod, R.M. and Orcutt, P. 1976. Dibutyryl Cyclic AMP, Adenosine and Guanosine Blockade of the Dopamine, Ergocryptine and Apomorphine Inhibition of Prolactin Release in Vitro. *Endocrinology* 99: 1612-1617.

Koga, H., *et al.* 2010. Successful treatment with mycophenolate mofetil of four Japanese patients with pemphigus vulgaris. *Eur J Dermatol*

20: 472-475.

Kulkarni, A.D. *et al.* 1994. The role of dietary sources of nucleotides in immune function: a review. *Journal of Nutrition*, 124: 1442S-1446S.

Lahita, R.G. (editor) *et al.* *Systemic Lupus Erythematosus*, Fifth Edition, 2011 Elsevier: New York.

Lee, M. *et al.* 2004. Mycophenolate mofetil in pyoderma gangrenosum. *J Dermatolog Treat* 15: 303-307.

Majithia, V. *et al.* 2005. Mycophenolate mofetil (CellCept): an alternative therapy for autoimmune inflammatory myopathy. *Rheumatology (Oxford)* 44: 386-389.

Navarro, J. *et al.* 1996. Modulation of antibody forming cell and mitogen driven lymphoproliferative responses by dietary nucleotides in mice. *Immunology Letters* 53: 141-145.

Nihtyanova, S.I. *et al.* 2007 Mycophenolate mofetil in diffuse cutaneous systemic sclerosis--a retrospective analysis. *Rheumatology (Oxford)*. 46:442-5.

Nikibakhsh, A.A., *et al.* 2010. Treatment of complicated Henoch-Schönlein Purpura with mycophenolate mofetil: a retrospective case series report. *Int J Rheumatol* 2010: 254316.

O'Connor, A.S. *et al.* 2003. Pancreatitis and duodenitis from sarcoidosis: successful therapy with mycophenolate mofetil. *Dig Dis Sci* 48: 2191-2195.

Pisoni, C. *et al.* 2007. Mycophenolate mofetil treatment in resistant myositis. *Rheumatology (Oxford)* 46: 516-518.

Rouster-Stevens, K. A. *et al.* 2010. Mycophenolate mofetil: a possible therapeutic agent for children with juvenile dermatomyositis.

Arthritis Care Res Hoboken 62: 1446-1451.

Saha, S. *et al.* 2011 Prolactin, Systemic Lupus Erythematosus, and autoreactive B cells: lessons learnt from murine models. *Clinical Reviews in Allergy and Immunology* 40: 8-15.

Sharzehi, K. *et al.* 2010. Mycophenolate mofetil for the treatment of autoimmune hepatitis in patients refractory or intolerant to conventional therapy. *Can J Gastroenterol* 24: 588-592.

Shelly, S. *et al.* H. 2012 Prolactin and Autoimmunity. *Autoimmunity Reviews* 11: A465-A470.

Ugrasbul, F. *et al.* 2008. Prevention of diabetes: effect of mycophenolate mofetil and anti-CD25 on onset of diabetes in the DRBB rat. *Pediatr Diabetes* 9: 596-601.

Yaniv G, *et al.* 2014. Volcanic explosion of autoantibodies in systemic Lupus erythematosus: A diversity of 180 different antibodies found in SLE patients. *Autoimmun Rev.* 2014 14:75-79.

Zhang, W. *et al.* 2005. Mycophenolate mofetil as a treatment for refractory idiopathic thrombocytopenic purpura. *Acta Pharmacol Sin* 26: 598-602.

About the Author
Steven A. Baranowitz, MD MS MBA

Dr. Steven A. Baranowitz is a physician and scientist with broad experience in dermatology, pharmaceutical new drug development, and biotechnology. He has extensive experience in both clinical practice and research. He was a medical director at several major pharmaceutical companies.

A graduate of the New York University School of Medicine, Dr. Baranowitz did his internship in Internal Medicine at Monmouth Medical Center in New Jersey. He then completed specialty training in Dermatology at Mount Sinai Hospital in New York and was also a Dermatology Research Fellow there. He obtained research experience in developmental biology while earning his Master of Science degree from the University of Michigan in Ann Arbor and his Bachelor of Science degree at Brooklyn College of the City University of New York. Dr. Baranowitz is an expert in pharmaceutical development of new medications, and received his M.B.A. at Fairleigh Dickinson University in Pharmaceutical and Chemical Studies.

Dr. Baranowitz has performed research at the University of Oxford in England, and at Oak Ridge National Laboratory in Oak Ridge, Tennessee. Dr. Baranowitz has presented papers at international symposia and his research has been published in scientific journals including the New England Journal of Medicine and the Journal of Theoretical Biology. He maintains a private dermatology practice in Narberth near Philadelphia, PA:

Steven Baranowitz, MD
145 N. Narberth Avenue
Narberth, PA 19072
610-660-9292
MyLupusDoc.com